MAKE YOUR OWN BATH BOMBS

A Guide to the Ins and Outs of Making Everyday Bubble Baths Even More Extraordinary

Disclaimer and Terms of Use:

Effort has been made to ensure that the information in this book is accurate and complete, however, the author and the publisher do not warrant the accuracy of the information, text and graphics contained within the book due to the rapidly changing nature of science, research, known and unknown facts and internet. The Author and the publisher do not hold any responsibility for errors, omissions or contrary interpretation of the subject matter herein. This book is presented solely for motivational and informational purposes only.

Table of Contents

Introduction: What Are Bath Bombs Exactly?

A long, luxurious bubble bath definitely counts as one of the most sublime pleasures in life, especially after a long day at work. Lying back and relaxing in a tub of soothing warm water while breathing in the wonderful scent of fragrant bath bubbles certainly does wonders for one's mood.

Up until recently, traditional baths were set up by merely strewing flower petals and herbs onto the bath water. Bottles of silky bubble bath liquid were added if the bather desired a foamy, fragrant bath. Bath bombs, however, blew both options out of the water when they were introduced to the market.

Primarily made up of a combination of weak acid and bicarbonate, bath bombs were designed to react to bath water by fizzing up vigorously as they dissolved, imbuing the bath with fragrance, color, bubbles, and the odd herb, flower petal, or glittering piece of confetti in the process. Although bath bombs are normally round, they can also be molded into more whimsical shapes like hearts or stars. Bath bombs can also be tinted with all sorts of colors in multiple combinations. Japanese versions of the quirky bath balls (called *bikkuri tamago*, or "surprise egg") even took things a step further by including miniature toys that were only revealed once the bath bomb was fully dissolved.

However, one primary drawback of bath bombs is that they are often good for only one use. Halving or dividing a bath ball can diminish its fizzing effectiveness as well as the overall effect (i.e., fragrance, bubbles) that it can impart upon the bath water. Another downside is that bath bombs are rather pricey, and many people hesitate to try them since buying and using one is virtually like throwing money down the drain.

Thus, the following recipes were compiled for the benefit of those who want to try the benefits of bath bombs without having to shell out a considerable amount of money. What's more is that much of the recipes in this book allow for multiple variations so avid bathers can customize the scent, color, and effect of their bath bombs to their hearts' content. The only limitation, as the cliché goes, is the maker's own creative imagination.

DIY Luxury: 25 Ways to Make Your Own Bath Bomb

Bath bombs are a bit trickier to make than their more common bath salts counterpart, and admittedly require more time to make since they need to be allowed to dry properly. Apart from including the basic ingredients that give bath bombs their fizz and permitting them to dry thoroughly before usage, there aren't really a lot of rules for making bath bombs. DIY enthusiasts fill find to their delight that the possibilities for adding scent, shaping, and tinting the charming bath fizz balls are virtually endless.

The primary ingredients (i.e., baking soda, Epsom salts) are readily available at most grocery stores while health and wellness stores often have wide and varied stocks of different essential oils. Citric acid is a bit harder to find, but a trip to the local pharmacy should fix that.

Some crafts stores do stock molds that were especially made for bath bombs, but a bit of ingenuity and resourcefulness could render their purchase unnecessary. Clean, empty plastic egg crates, ice cube trays, muffin trays, and even plastic Easter eggs (the sort that come in halves) will do very nicely as molds for homemade bath bombs.

Lastly, while each recipe generally indicates which essential oil to use, substitutions and variations can be made (depending on the purpose of the bath bomb). Below is a list of a few common essential oils and their health and/or well-being benefits:

- Lavender: excellent for relaxation and for aiding sleep

- Green tea/citrus: ideal for invigorating the senses

- Cinnamon/vanilla: lush and rich, these heavy scents are great for establishing a sensual, amorous mood

- Ginger: can aid in clearing the mind and sharpening one's focus

- Chamomile: calming and relaxing, can also bring about a restful night's sleep

Traditional Bath Bomb

Perhaps the most basic bath bomb recipe, this can be the base for a variety of bath bombs with different shapes, colors, scents, and additives. Matching the food coloring to the essential oil used (e.g., purple for lavender, green for fresh grass or tea, etc.) is highly advised.

Ingredients

1 cup baking soda

¾ cup cornstarch

½ cup citric acid (in powder form, not liquid. As a substitute, citric acid tablets can be ground up to make a powder)

Water

Food coloring (in gel or liquid form)

Essential oil/s of choice (about 8-10 drops)

Directions

1. In a metal or glass bowl, mix together baking soda, cornstarch, and citric acid powder. (Using one's hands is preferable since this gives one a better feel for the mixture.)

2. Add the water in, a drop at a time. (An eye dropper or an atomizer bottle can be used in this step to control the amount of water added.) Enough water has been added when the mixture is moist enough to form into dough. Be wary of adding too much water as this will cause the mixture to turn mushy.

3. Add in the food coloring and the essential oils, mixing thoroughly after each addition. Note that a little bit of food coloring goes a long way, so it is better to add such gradually.

4. Portion the bath bomb mixture and press into the molds. The mixture must be pressed firmly into the molds to prevent any air from entering the bath bomb. (Excess air can cause the bath bomb to crack and break.)

5. Leave the mixture to dry in the molds for at least 24 hours. This will ensure that the mixture will hold its shape. However, if the bath bombs are still damp to the touch after 24 hours, they may be carefully taken out of the molds and allowed to air dry on a clean towel.

Skin-Softening Bath Bombs

As their name suggests, these bath bombs have the added benefit of moisturizing and softening skin. Thus, bath salts and food coloring are omitted from this recipe as they can have a drying effect on skin. Argan oil can also be substituted for the sweet almond oil for a luxurious touch.

Ingredients

1 cup cornstarch

½ cup baking soda

½ cup citric acid powder

¼ cup shea butter

6 tablespoons sweet almond oil

8-10 drops of essential oil (vanilla or cinnamon is advised for this bath bomb)

Directions

1. In a metal or glass bowl, stir together all the dry ingredients until well-mixed.

2. Mix together the wet ingredients (shea butter, sweet almond oil, and essential oils), and then add them to the dry ingredients. Mix well.

3. Using the hands, form the mixture into balls and firmly stuff them into the molds, making sure that no air enters the mixture.

4. Allow the mixture to dry for 24 hours, and then unmold onto clean dry towels to dry for a longer period of time if needed.

Lavender Flower Bombs

Lavender is a popular scent for bath bombs due to its role as a sleep aid. The intricate baking tin used as a mold for these bombs give them their distinctive floral shape.

Ingredients

1 cup baking soda

¾ cup cornstarch

½ cup citric acid powder

Water

Red and blue food coloring (in gel or liquid form)

5 drops of lavender essential oil

Directions

1. In a metal or glass bowl, stir together all the dry ingredients until well-mixed.

2. Fill a small atomizer bottle with about ¼ cup water, and then add about 5-8 drops of red food coloring. Shake well to mix. Do the same for the blue food coloring.

3. Spray the dry mixture with the food coloring, alternating the red and blue colors. Mix well after each addition, and stop spraying once the desired hue is reached.

4. Add the lavender essential oils and mix well until the entire mixture is scented.

5. Using the hands, form the mixture into balls and firmly stuff them into a mini bundt baking tin, making sure that no air enters the mixture.

6. Allow the mixture to dry for 24 hours, and then unmold very carefully onto clean dry towels to dry for a longer period of time if needed.

Peppermint Bath Tablets

Peppermint essential oils are known to have an invigorating and rejuvenating effect on the senses. Peppermint is also known to help clear one's airways in the event of a cold or a stuffy nose.

These bath tablets take their shape from flat muffin tins, which are common enough in any household kitchen.

Ingredients

1 cup baking soda

¾ cup cornstarch

½ cup citric acid powder

Water

Green food coloring (in gel or liquid form)

5 to 7 drops of peppermint essential oil

Directions

1. In a metal or glass bowl, stir together all the dry ingredients until well-mixed.

2. Fill a small atomizer bottle with about ¼ cup water, and then add about 5-8 drops of green food coloring. Shake well to mix.

3. Spray the dry mixture with the food coloring, mixing well after each addition, up until the desired hue is reached.

4. Add the peppermint essential oils (5 drops is enough to give it a distinct peppermint scent, but up to 7 drops can increase the intensity if the peppermint bath is meant to open up the sinuses) and mix well until the entire mixture is scented.

5. Using the hands, form the mixture into balls and firmly stuff them into a flat muffin baking tin, making sure that no air enters the mixture.

6. Allow the mixture to dry for 24 hours, and then unmold very carefully onto clean dry towels to dry for a longer period of time if needed.

Pink Grapefruit Bath Eggs

Blush pink, petite, and egg-like, these fresh and citrusy bath bombs would make wonderful Easter giveaways.

Ingredients

1 cup baking soda

¾ cup cornstarch

½ cup citric acid powder

Water

Red food coloring (in gel or liquid form)

6 to 7 drops of grapefruit essential oil

Directions

1. In a metal or glass bowl, stir together all the dry ingredients until well-mixed.

2. Fill a small atomizer bottle with about ¼ cup water, and then add about 4-6 drops of green food coloring (4 drops will result in a baby pink hue while 6 drops will result in a fuchsia tint). Shake well to mix.

3. Spray the dry mixture with the food coloring, mixing well after each addition, up until the desired hue is reached.

4. Add the grapefruit essential oils and mix well until the entire mixture is scented.

5. Using the hands, form the mixture into balls and firmly stuff them into the halves of plastic Easter eggs, making sure that no air enters the mixture. Carefully bring the two Easter egg halves together and twist to secure.

6. Allow the mixture to dry for 24 hours, and then unmold very carefully onto clean dry towels to dry for a longer period of time if needed.

Autumn Leaf Bath Bombs

These autumn-hued bath bombs are infused with the heady scents of cinnamon, clove, and orange essential oils. Leaf-shaped bath bomb molds can be purchased at most crafts stores.

Ingredients

1 cup baking soda

¾ cup cornstarch

½ cup citric acid powder

Water

Red and yellow food coloring (in gel or liquid form)

3 drops of cinnamon essential oil

3 drops of clove essential oil

3 drops of orange essential oil

Directions

1. In a metal or glass bowl, stir together all the dry ingredients until well-mixed.

2. Fill a small atomizer bottle with about ¼ cup water, and then add about 5 drops of red food coloring. Shake well to mix. Do the same for the yellow food coloring

3. Spray the dry mixture with the food coloring (alternating between the red and yellow food coloring mixes). Mix well after each addition, up until the desired hue (a mellow orange) is reached.

4. Combine the cinnamon, clove, and orange essential oils together and stir them into the entire mixture.

5. Using the hands, form the mixture into balls and firmly stuff them into the plastic leaf molds.

6. Allow the mixture to dry for 24 hours, and then unmold very carefully onto clean dry towels to dry for a longer period of time if needed.

Fresh Tea and Bamboo Bath Leaves

With their fresh, clean scents, these leaf-like bath bombs are great for an invigorating bath.

Ingredients

1 cup baking soda

¾ cup cornstarch

½ cup citric acid powder

Water

Green and yellow food coloring (in gel or liquid form)

5 drops of lemon essential oils

7 drops of green tea essential oils

5 drops of fresh bamboo essential oils

Directions

1. In a metal or glass bowl, stir together all the dry ingredients until well-mixed.

2. Fill a small atomizer bottle with about ¼ cup water, and then add about 5 drops of green food coloring. Shake well to mix. Do the same for the yellow food coloring

3. Spray the dry mixture with the food coloring (alternating between the green and yellow food coloring mixes). Mix well after each addition, up until the desired hue (a vibrant, leafy green) is reached.

4. Combine the lemon, green tea and fresh bamboo essential oils together and stir them into the entire mixture.

5. Using the hands, form the mixture into balls and firmly stuff them into the plastic leaf molds.

6. Allow the mixture to dry for 24 hours, and then unmold very carefully onto clean dry towels to dry for a longer period of time if needed.

Jasmine Flower Bombs

These bath bombs make ideal party souvenirs (especially for bridal showers or birthday parties) due to its pretty powder yellow color and its luscious jasmine fragrance. Dried jasmine flowers are added to give this recipe more oomph.

Ingredients

1 cup baking soda

½ cup citric acid powder

½ cup cornstarch

½ cup Epsom salts or bath salts

Water

Yellow food coloring (in gel or liquid form)

Jasmine essential oil

½ cup dried jasmine flowers

Plastic flower head, preferably in a matching hue (these can be purchased cheaply in bulk from certain flower shops)

Directions

1. Mix the baking soda, citric acid powder, and cornstarch in a bowl. Using a sieve, carefully sift the powder to ensure that there are no lumps. Stir in the bath salts.

2. Fill a small atomizer bottle with about ¼ cup water, and then add about 5 drops of yellow food coloring. Shake well to mix.

3. Spray the dry mixture with the food coloring, mixing well after each addition, up until a powdery yellow hue is reached.

4. Stir in about 6-8 drops of the jasmine essential oils, along with the dried jasmine flowers.

5. Using the hands, form the mixture around the plastic flower heads, making a ball with the flower head peeking out from the top.

6. Pack the mixture into circular molds and leave to dry for 24 hours, and then unmold very carefully onto clean dry towels. These may be wrapped individually in clear cellophane bags as giveaways.

Rose Oil Bath Cubes

Rose oil is a timeless fragrance, and a sprinkling of dried rosemary herbs gives these bath cubes an added earthiness.

Ingredients

¼ cup citric acid powder

½ cup baking powder

Water

Red food coloring (in gel or liquid form)

Rose oil

3 tablespoons dried rosemary

Directions

1. Mix the citric acid powder and baking soda in a bowl.

2. Fill a small atomizer bottle with about ¼ cup water, and then add about 5 drops of red food coloring. Shake well to mix.

3. Spray the dry mixture with the food coloring, mixing well after each addition, up until a bright pink hue is reached.

4. Stir in about 6 drops of the rose oils, along with the dried rosemary.

5. Pack the mixture into a clean plastic ice cube tray and leave to dry for 24 hours, and then unmold very carefully onto clean dry towels.

Mint Chocolate Bath Pastilles

Sweet-smelling and decadent, these bath bombs also contain a milky component which softens the skin.

Ingredients

1 cup baking soda

1 cup citric acid

½ cup cornstarch

½ cup powdered milk

Water

Green food coloring

3 tablespoons cocoa butter

4 drops peppermint essential oil

¼ cup dried cacao nibs, finely chopped

Directions

1. In a metal or glass bowl, stir together all the dry ingredients until well-mixed.

2. Fill a small atomizer bottle with about ¼ cup water, and then add about 5 drops of green food coloring. Shake well to mix.

3. Spray the dry mixture with the food coloring, mixing well after each addition, up until the desired hue (a light, powdery green) is reached.

4. Stir in the cocoa butter, along with the peppermint oils, mixing well until the entire mixture is scented.

5. Add the dried cacao nibs, stirring well to incorporate them into the mixture.

6. Using the hands, form the mixture into balls and firmly stuff them into a flat muffin baking tin, making sure that no air enters the mixture.

7. Allow the mixture to dry for 24 hours, and then unmold very carefully onto clean dry towels to dry for a longer period of time if needed.

Glittering Bergamot Bath Eggs

As an alternative to the girly pink grapefruit bath eggs, these bergamot eggs have a stronger citrus scent and even impart a bit of glimmer to the bath water.

Ingredients

1 cup baking soda

¾ cup cornstarch

½ cup citric acid powder

Water

Yellow food coloring (in gel or liquid form)

6-7 drops of bergamot essential oil

Cosmetic glitter

Directions

1. In a metal or glass bowl, stir together all the dry ingredients until well-mixed.

2. Fill a small atomizer bottle with about ¼ cup water, and then add about 8 drops of yellow food coloring. Shake well to mix.

3. Spray the dry mixture with the food coloring, mixing well after each addition, up until the desired hue (a vibrant bright yellow) is reached.

4. Add the bergamot essential oils and mix well until the entire mixture is scented. Stir in the cosmetic glitter, making sure that it is well distributed throughout the mixture.

5. Using the hands, form the mixture into balls and firmly stuff them into the halves of plastic Easter eggs, making sure that no air enters the mixture. Carefully bring the two Easter egg halves together and twist to secure.

6. Allow the mixture to dry for 24 hours, and then unmold very carefully onto clean dry towels to dry for a longer period of time if needed.

Mini Lavender Sleep Bombs

Since long baths before going to bed aren't always an option, these mini bath bombs allow for a quick but still relaxing soak.

Ingredients

½ cup citric acid

1 cup baking soda

½ cup cornstarch

Water

Red and blue food coloring (in gel or liquid form)

Olive oil

5 drops of lavender essential oil

Directions

1. Mix the dry ingredients in a bowl.

2. Fill a small atomizer bottle with about ¼ cup water, and then add about 5 drops of red food coloring. Shake well to mix. Do the same for the blue food coloring

3. Spray the dry mixture with the food coloring, alternating between the red and the blue food coloring mixture. Mix well after each addition, up until a light purple hue is reached.

4. Stir in about a tablespoon of the olive oil, along with the lavender oil.

5. Pack the mixture into a clean plastic ice cube tray and leave to dry for 24 hours, and then unmold very carefully onto clean dry towels.

Mini Citrus Energy Bombs

While the lavender mini bombs are for inducing sleep, these citrusy bombs are best for a brief pick-me-up at the beginning of a long work day.

Since long baths before going to bed aren't always an option, these mini bath bombs allow for a quick but still relaxing soak.

Ingredients

½ cup citric acid

1 cup baking soda

½ cup cornstarch

Water

Green and yellow food coloring (in gel or liquid form)

Olive oil

3 drops of lemon essential oil

6 drops of bergamot essential oil

Directions

1. Mix the dry ingredients in a bowl.

2. Fill a small atomizer bottle with about ¼ cup water, and then add about 5 drops of green food coloring. Shake well to mix. Do the same for the yellow food coloring

3. Spray the dry mixture with the food coloring, alternating between the green and the yellow food coloring mixture. Mix well after each addition, up until a bright yellow-green hue is reached.

4. Stir in about a tablespoon of the olive oil, along with the lemon and bergamot essential oils.

5. Pack the mixture into a clean plastic ice cube tray and leave to dry for 24 hours, and then unmold very carefully onto clean dry towels.

Chamomile Flower Bombs

This variation on the lavender flower bombs uses chamomile, a fragrant flower that offers similar sleep aid benefits. Vanilla essential oils are added to mellow out the fragrance mix.

Ingredients

1 cup baking soda

¾ cup cornstarch

½ cup citric acid powder

Water

Yellow food coloring (in gel or liquid form)

3 drops of vanilla essential oils

4 drops of chamomile essential oils

Directions

1. In a metal or glass bowl, stir together all the dry ingredients until well-mixed.

2. Fill a small atomizer bottle with about ¼ cup water, and then add about 7 drops of yellow food coloring. Shake well to mix.

3. Spray the dry mixture with the yellow food coloring, mixing well after each addition. A light, dusty yellow is the desired color.

4. Combine the chamomile and vanilla essential oils and stir into the mixture until it is thoroughly scented.

5. Using the hands, form the mixture into balls and firmly stuff them into a mini bundt baking tin, making sure that no air enters the mixture.

6. Allow the mixture to dry for 24 hours, and then unmold very carefully onto clean dry towels to dry for a longer period of time if needed.

Cinnamon Bath Hearts

Perfect for Valentine's Day, these heart-shaped bath bombs leave the bath water mildly scented with cinnamon and rose oil, perfect for a romantic interlude.

Ingredients

1 cup baking soda

Half a cup of cornstarch

1 cup citric acid

Water

Red food coloring

3 tablespoons cocoa butter

4 drops cinnamon essential oil

3 drops rose oil

Directions

1. In a metal or glass bowl, stir together all the dry ingredients until well-mixed.

2. Fill a small atomizer bottle with about ¼ cup water, and then add about 5 drops of red food coloring. Shake well to mix.

3. Spray the dry mixture with the food coloring, mixing well after each addition, up until the desired hue (a deep pink) is reached.

4. Stir in the cocoa butter, along with the cinnamon and rose oils, mixing well until the entire mixture is scented.

5. Using the hands, form the mixture into balls and firmly stuff them into heart-shaped molds, making sure that no air enters the mixture.

6. Allow the mixture to dry for 24 hours, and then unmold very carefully onto clean dry towels to dry for a longer period of time if needed.

Vanilla Bergamot Bath Tablets

Imparting both comforting warmth and uplifting freshness to one's bath, these bath bombs are as beneficial (and perhaps even more so) to one's health as the medicine that they resemble.

Ingredients

1 cup baking soda

Half a cup of cornstarch

1 cup citric acid

Water

3 drops vanilla essential oil

5 drops bergamot essential oil

Dried vanilla bean husks

Directions

1. In a metal or glass bowl, stir together all the dry ingredients until well-mixed.

2. Slowly add in water, drop by drop, into the mixture until it forms a ball of dough.

3. Combine the vanilla and bergamot essential oils, and stir into the mixture.

4. Portion the dried vanilla bean husks into each of the openings of the flat muffin tin, making sure that each piece is right smack in the middle of the circle.

5. Using the hands, form the mixture into balls and firmly stuff them into a flat muffin baking tin, making sure that no air enters the mixture.

6. Allow the mixture to dry for 24 hours, and then unmold very carefully onto clean dry towels to dry for a longer period of time if needed.

Clarifying Rosemary Bath Lozenges

The rosemary herb is prized for its clarifying aroma, and its ability to clear the mind. Thus, these lozenges can produce a bath to wash away all the worries and stress of a hectic work week.

Ingredients

1 cup baking soda

Half a cup of cornstarch

1 cup citric acid

Water

3 drops lemon essential oil

5 drops rosemary essential oil

3 tablespoons dried rosemary leaves

Directions

1. In a metal or glass bowl, stir together all the dry ingredients until well-mixed.

2. Slowly add in water, drop by drop, into the mixture until it forms a ball of dough.

3. Combine the lemon and rosemary essential oils, and stir into the mixture.

4. Stir in the dried rosemary leaves into the mixture.

5. Using the hands, form the mixture into balls and firmly stuff them into a flat muffin baking tin, making sure that no air enters the mixture.

6. Allow the mixture to dry for 24 hours, and then unmold very carefully onto clean dry towels to dry for a longer period of time if needed.

Spicy Confetti Bath Bombs

Though the bits of cosmetic glitter and confetti don't really add any fragrance or medicinal value to this bath bomb, they do add a festive touch to this cheery bath ball.

Ingredients

1 cup baking soda

½ cup citric acid powder

½ cup cornstarch

½ cup Epsom salts or bath salts

Water

Yellow and red food coloring (in gel or liquid form)

3 drops ylang-ylang essential oil

3 drops ginger essential oil

4 drops sandalwood essential oil

¼ cup cosmetic glitter

¼ cup confetti

Directions

1. Mix the dry ingredients together in a bowl.

2. Fill a small atomizer bottle with about ¼ cup water, and then add about 5 drops of yellow food coloring. Shake well to mix. Do the same for the red food coloring

3. Spray the dry mixture with the food coloring, mixing well after each addition, up until a flame orange hue is reached.

4. Combine the ylang-ylang, ginger, and sandalwood essential oils, and stir into the mixture. Mix in the cosmetic glitter and confetti.

5. Pack the mixture into plastic circular molds and leave to dry for 24 hours, and then unmold very carefully onto clean dry towels.

Oriental Flower Bombs

With their rustic, woody scents, these reddish flowers lend a wonderful sensuality to everyday bathwater.

Ingredients

1 cup baking soda

¾ cup cornstarch

½ cup citric acid powder

Water

Red food coloring (in gel or liquid form)

5 drops of jasmine essential oil

3 drops of sandalwood essential oil

3 drops of ylang-ylang essential oil

Directions

1. In a metal or glass bowl, stir together all the dry ingredients until well-mixed.

2. Fill a small atomizer bottle with about ¼ cup water, and then add about 5-8 drops of red food coloring. Shake well to mix.

3. Spray the dry mixture with the food coloring, mixing well after each addition. A vivid red hue is preferred.

4. Combine the jasmine, sandalwood, and ylang-ylang essential oils and stir them in until the entire mixture is scented.

5. Using the hands, form the mixture into balls and firmly stuff them into a mini bundt baking tin, making sure that no air enters the mixture.

6. Allow the mixture to dry for 24 hours, and then unmold very carefully onto clean dry towels to dry for a longer period of time if needed.

Lemon Lavender Bath Pastilles

Though they are guaranteed show-stoppers, these dual color bath bombs are actually quite easy to make.

Ingredients

1 cup baking soda

1 cup citric acid

½ cup cornstarch

Water

Yellow, red, and blue food coloring (in gel or liquid form)

3 drops lemon essential oil

5 drops lavender essential oil

Directions

1. In a metal or glass bowl, stir together all the dry ingredients until well-mixed. Divide the mixture evenly into two bowls.

2. Using a small atomizer, combine ¼ cup of water and about five drops of yellow food coloring. Shake well to combine. Do the same for the red and blue food coloring.

3. Spray one half of the dry mixture with the red and blue food coloring, alternating between the colors and mixing well after each addition, until a light purple color is achieved. Stir in the lavender essential oils.

4. Spray the other half of the dry mixture with the yellow food coloring, mixing well after each addition, until a dusty yellow color is achieved. Stir in the lemon essential oils.

5. Using the hands, place the purple mixture into the halves of a flat muffin pan's receptacles. Place the yellow mixture into the other halves. Press the mixtures firmly together, eliminating any excess air.

6. Allow the mixture to dry for 24 hours, and then unmold very carefully onto clean dry towels to dry for a longer period of time if needed.

Peppermint Candy Bath Bombs

What's Christmas without those peppermint candy canes? This recipe uses a special candy cane mold to bring the holidays to one's bathtub.

Ingredients

1 cup citric acid

1 cup baking soda

½ cup cornstarch

5 drops peppermint essential oil

Water

Red food coloring (in gel or liquid form)

Directions

1. In a metal or glass bowl, stir together all the dry ingredients until well-mixed. Add in the peppermint essential oils. Divide the mixture evenly into two bowls.

2. Using a small atomizer, combine ¼ cup of water and about five drops of red food coloring. Shake well to combine.

3. Spray one half of the dry mixture with the red food coloring, mixing well after each addition, until a light pink color is achieved.

4. Using the hands, place lumps of the pink and white mixture into the candy cane molds, forming alternate stripes. Press firmly into the mold to block out any excess air.

5. Allow the mixture to dry for 24 hours, and then unmold onto clean dry towels to dry for a longer period of time if needed.

"Gingerbread" Star Bombs

Infused with ginger, cinnamon, and clove essential oils, these star-shaped bath balls bring to mind the nostalgia of a child's gingerbread house during the holidays.

Ingredients

1 cup baking soda

¾ cup cornstarch

½ cup citric acid powder

Water

Red and yellow food coloring (in gel or liquid form)

3 drops of cinnamon essential oil

4 drops of clove essential oil

5 drops of ginger essential oil

Directions

1. In a metal or glass bowl, stir together all the dry ingredients until well-mixed.

2. Fill a small atomizer bottle with about ¼ cup water, and then add about 5 drops of red food coloring. Shake well to mix. Do the same for the yellow food coloring.

3. Spray the dry mixture with the food coloring (alternating between the red and yellow food coloring mixes). Mix well after each addition, up until the desired hue (a bright orange) is reached.

4. Combine the cinnamon, clove, and ginger essential oils together and stir them into the entire mixture.

5. Using the hands, form the mixture into balls and firmly stuff them into the plastic star molds.

6. Allow the mixture to dry for 24 hours, and then unmold very carefully onto clean dry towels to dry for a longer period of time if needed.

Ginger Tea Bath Capsules

Ginger, green tea, and fresh bamboo come together in this bright, zesty tonic to uplift the senses.

Ingredients

1 cup baking soda

1 cup citric acid

Half a cup of cornstarch

Water

Yellow and green food coloring (in gel or liquid form)

5 drops ginger essential oil

6 drops fresh bamboo essential oil

7 drops green tea essential oil

Directions

1. In a metal or glass bowl, stir together all the dry ingredients until well-mixed. Divide the mixture evenly into two bowls.

2. Using a small atomizer, combine ¼ cup of water and about seven drops of yellow food coloring. Shake well to combine. Do the same for the green food coloring.

3. Spray one half of the dry mixture with the yellow food coloring, mixing well after each addition, until a vibrant yellow color is achieved. Stir in the ginger essential oils.

4. Spray the other half of the dry mixture with the green food coloring, mixing well after each addition, until a bright leaf-green color is achieved. Stir in the fresh bamboo and green tea essential oils.

5. Using the hands, place the yellow mixture into the halves of a plastic Easter egg. Place the green mixture into the other halves. Press the plastic halves firmly together, eliminating any excess air.

6. Allow the mixture to dry for 24 hours, and then unmold very carefully onto clean dry towels to dry for a longer period of time if needed.

Lavender Ylang-Ylang Bath Hearts

The soft fragrance of the ylang-ylang is a perfect foil to the earthiness of the lavender blossoms, and this bath bomb features the best of both.

Ingredients

1 cup baking soda

1 cup citric acid

Half a cup of cornstarch

Water

5 drops lavender essential oil

5 drops ylang-ylang essential oil

3 tablespoons dried lavender blossoms

2 tablespoons dried ylang-ylang blossoms

Directions

1. In a metal or glass bowl, stir together all the dry ingredients until well-mixed.

2. Add the water in to the mixture, drop by drop, until it becomes moist enough to form a ball of dough.

3. Combine the lavender and ylang-ylang essential oils, and stir into the mixture. Add in the dried blossoms.

4. Using the hands, form the mixture into balls and firmly stuff them into heart-shaped molds, making sure that no air enters the mixture.

5. Allow the mixture to dry for 24 hours, and then unmold very carefully onto clean dry towels to dry for a longer period of time if needed.

Citrus Peppermint Pick-Me-Up Easter Eggs

With their bright yellow and pink colors (as well as their perky, clean scent), these grown-up Easter eggs are sure-fire crowd pleasers.

Ingredients

1 cup baking soda

1 cup citric acid

Half a cup of cornstarch

Water

Yellow and red food coloring (in gel or liquid form)

5 drops peppermint essential oil

6 drops lemon essential oil

3 drops orange essential oil

Directions

1. In a metal or glass bowl, stir together all the dry ingredients until well-mixed. Divide the mixture evenly into two bowls.

2. Using a small atomizer, combine ¼ cup of water and about five drops of yellow food coloring. Shake well to combine. Do the same for the red food coloring.

3. Spray one half of the dry mixture with the red food coloring, mixing well after each addition, until a blush pink color is achieved. Stir in the peppermint oils.

4. Spray the other half of the dry mixture with the yellow food coloring, mixing well after each addition, until a dusty yellow color is achieved. Stir in the lemon and orange essential oils.

5. Using the hands, place the yellow mixture into the halves of a plastic Easter egg. Place the pink mixture into the other halves. Press the plastic halves firmly together, eliminating any excess air.

6. Allow the mixture to dry for 24 hours, and then unmold very carefully onto clean dry towels to dry for a longer period of time if needed.

Conclusion: A Few Reminders on the Care and Keeping of Bath Bombs

As with anything that comes in to direct contact with bare skin, bath bombs do have the potential to cause skin allergies or irritation. To avoid such, make sure to conduct a patch test prior to adding any substances to the bath bomb base mixture. To do this, take a few drops of the said additive and apply to the inner crease of the elbow. Should a great deal of time pass (say about 24 hours), and the skin remains free of any redness or rashes, it would be safe to include the additive into the bath bomb.

Bath salts are often a key ingredient in many bath bombs. The expensive kinds might up the luxury quotient of both the bath bomb and the bathing experience it creates, but caution should be exercised in the amount of bath salts added since they can be rather drying to the skin.

Cornstarch is also a popular component for homemade bath bombs since their chemical composition enables the bath balls to float while they fizz away. However, women with pre-existing yeast infections should refrain from adding cornstarch to their bath bombs since they can aggravate the infection.

It should also be noted that bath bombs, especially homemade ones, are very sensitive to damp or humid climates. Thus, it is crucial to keep them dry prior to usage. And while it might seem intuitive to store bath bombs in the bathroom, doing so is not advisable if the room also contains a sauna or is often flooded with a great deal of steam on a regular basis (the moist vapors could cause the bath balls to collapse).

Lastly, bath bombs should not be stored away for too long as any essential oils scenting them could evaporate and thus render them nothing more than colored fizzy bath powder. After all, although bath bombs are undoubtedly a treat to use, one can and should always find a reason to indulge in a bath at any given time.